EPI DIET MEAL PLAN

Nourishing Solutions for Exocrine Pancreatic Insufficiency (EPI) through Tailored Meal Plans and Wholesome Recipes

DR. Dorothy Cline

Copyright © 2024

All Rights Are Reserved

The content in this book may not be reproduced, duplicated, or transferred without the express written permission of the author or publisher. Under no circumstances will the publisher or author be held liable or legally responsible for any losses, expenditures, or damages incurred directly or indirectly as a consequence of the information included in this book.

Legal Remarks

Copyright protection applies to this publication. It is only intended for personal use. No piece of this work may be modified, distributed, sold, quoted, or paraphrased without the author's or publisher's consent.

Disclaimer Statement

Please keep in mind that the contents of this booklet are meant for educational and recreational purposes. Every effort has been made to offer accurate, up-to-date, reliable, and thorough information. There are, however, no stated or implied assurances of any kind. Readers understand that the author is providing competent counsel. The content in this book originates from several sources. Please seek the opinion of a Stop Storing Fat, Balance Hormones and Lose Weight Naturally by Eating More Food Through Delicious Recipes and just 7 days Meal Plan

competent professional before using any of the tactics outlined in this book. By reading this book, the reader agrees that the author will not be held accountable for any direct or indirect damages resulting from the use of the information contained therein, including, but not limited to, errors, omissions, or inaccuracies.

TABLE OF CONTENTS

Chapter 1 4
Introduction to the EPI Diet Meal Plan 4
Chapter 2 9
Understanding EPI (Exocrine Pancreatic Insufficiency) 9
Chapter 3 13
Basics of the EPI Diet 13
Chapter 4 17
Creating Your EPI Diet Meal Plan 17
    Calculating Caloric Needs 17
    Determining Macronutrient Ratios 19
    Meal Planning Strategies 22
Chapter 5 26
Sample Meal Plans 26
    Beginner's Week Meal Plan 26
    Intermediate Week Meal Plan 35
    Advanced Week Meal Plan 46
Chapter 6 58
Recipes for EPI Diet Meals 58
    Breakfast Recipes 58
    Lunch Recipes 67
    Dinner Recipes 76
    Snack Recipes 88
Conclusion 96

CHAPTER 1

INTRODUCTION TO THE EPI DIET MEAL PLAN

In today's fast-paced world, where convenience often trumps nutrition, many individuals find themselves struggling with various health challenges. Among these challenges is Exocrine Pancreatic Insufficiency (EPI), a condition that affects the pancreas's ability to produce necessary enzymes for proper digestion. EPI can lead to malabsorption of nutrients, weight loss, and a host of gastrointestinal symptoms, profoundly impacting one's quality of life.

Understanding the gravity of managing EPI, individuals seek effective strategies to navigate their dietary needs while maintaining optimal health. The EPI Diet Meal Plan emerges as a beacon of hope, offering a structured approach to nutrition tailored specifically to address the unique requirements of individuals with EPI.

In this comprehensive guide, we embark on a journey to explore the intricacies of the EPI Diet Meal Plan, delving into its foundations, practical applications, and the transformative impact it can have on those grappling with EPI.

Unveiling the Essence of the EPI Diet Meal Plan

At its core, the EPI Diet Meal Plan is designed to support individuals with EPI in optimizing their nutritional intake while minimizing digestive distress. It emphasizes consuming foods rich in essential nutrients while being mindful of the digestive limitations posed by EPI. By strategically selecting foods that are easily digestible and well-tolerated, individuals can mitigate symptoms and enhance their overall well-being.

Navigating the Landscape of EPI

Before delving into the specifics of the EPI Diet Meal Plan, it's crucial to gain a deeper understanding of EPI itself. Exocrine Pancreatic Insufficiency occurs when the pancreas fails to produce adequate enzymes, such as lipase, protease, and amylase, necessary for breaking down fats, proteins, and carbohydrates, respectively. As a result, individuals with EPI often experience difficulties digesting food, leading to nutrient malabsorption and related complications.

The Pillars of the EPI Diet

The EPI Diet Meal Plan rests upon several fundamental principles aimed at optimizing nutrition while accommodating the digestive challenges associated with EPI:

Balanced Nutrition: The EPI Diet emphasizes a balanced intake of macronutrients, including carbohydrates, proteins, and fats, tailored to meet individual needs while supporting overall health and well-being.

Digestive Support: Given the compromised digestive function in EPI, the diet prioritizes easily digestible foods and incorporates enzyme replacement therapy as necessary to aid in the digestion and absorption of nutrients.

Nutrient Density: Maximizing the nutritional value of each meal is paramount in the EPI Diet. Emphasis is placed on incorporating nutrient-dense foods rich in vitamins, minerals, and antioxidants to support optimal health and vitality.

Meal Timing and Frequency: Consistent meal timing and appropriate meal frequency play a crucial role in managing EPI symptoms and stabilizing blood sugar levels. The EPI Diet advocates for regular, balanced meals and snacks throughout the day to support optimal digestion and nutrient absorption.

Crafting Your EPI Diet Meal Plan

Building an effective EPI Diet Meal Plan requires careful consideration of individual needs, preferences, and dietary restrictions. Key steps in crafting a personalized meal plan include:

Assessing Nutritional Requirements: Determining caloric needs and macronutrient ratios based on factors such as age, gender, activity level, and metabolic status lays the foundation for an effective meal plan.

Selecting Suitable Foods: Identifying foods that are well-tolerated and easily digestible is essential in creating a meal plan that supports optimal digestion and nutrient absorption.

Creating Balanced Meals: Structuring meals to include a combination of lean proteins, complex carbohydrates, healthy fats, and fiber-rich foods ensures a balanced nutritional profile and sustained energy levels throughout the day.

Incorporating Variety and Flavor: Exploring diverse culinary options and incorporating a variety of flavors, textures, and cooking methods adds excitement and enjoyment to the EPI Diet Meal Plan, making it sustainable in the long term.

Embracing a Journey to Wellness

Embarking on the EPI Diet Meal Plan journey is not merely about managing symptoms; it's about reclaiming control over one's health and embracing a lifestyle centered around nourishment, vitality, and well-being. With dedication, mindfulness, and a commitment to self-care, individuals with EPI can unlock the transformative power of nutrition and embark on a path to wellness.

CHAPTER 2

UNDERSTANDING EPI (EXOCRINE PANCREATIC INSUFFICIENCY)

Exocrine Pancreatic Insufficiency (EPI) is a complex gastrointestinal disorder characterized by the inadequate production or secretion of digestive enzymes by the pancreas. These essential enzymes, including lipase, protease, and amylase, play a crucial role in breaking down fats, proteins, and carbohydrates, respectively, facilitating their absorption in the small intestine.

The Role of the Pancreas

The pancreas is a vital organ situated behind the stomach in the abdomen. It serves a dual function as both an endocrine and exocrine gland. While its endocrine function involves the secretion of hormones such as insulin and glucagon, which regulate blood sugar levels, its exocrine function is primarily focused on producing digestive enzymes essential for proper digestion and nutrient absorption.

Causes of EPI

EPI can arise from various underlying conditions or factors that impair the pancreas's ability to produce or deliver digestive enzymes to the small intestine. Some common **causes of EPI include:**

- Chronic Pancreatitis: Prolonged inflammation of the pancreas can lead to irreversible damage to the pancreatic tissue, resulting in diminished enzyme production.
- Cystic Fibrosis: Individuals with cystic fibrosis often experience thickened mucus that can obstruct the pancreatic ducts, impairing the release of digestive enzymes into the intestines.
- Pancreatic Surgery or Trauma: Surgical procedures involving the pancreas or traumatic injuries to the abdomen can disrupt the normal functioning of the pancreas, leading to EPI.
- Autoimmune Conditions: Autoimmune disorders such as autoimmune pancreatitis can cause inflammation and damage to the pancreatic tissue, impairing enzyme secretion.
- Genetic Factors: Inherited genetic mutations affecting the pancreas's structure or function can predispose individuals to develop EPI.

Signs and Symptoms

The symptoms of EPI can vary in severity depending on the degree of enzyme deficiency and the underlying cause. Common signs and symptoms of EPI may include:

- Steatorrhea: Excessive fat in the stool, leading to greasy, foul-smelling stools.
- Weight Loss: Inadequate digestion and absorption of nutrients can result in unintended weight loss and malnutrition.
- Abdominal Pain: Discomfort or pain in the abdominal region, often associated with bloating and gas.
- Nutritional Deficiencies: Deficiencies in fat-soluble vitamins (A, D, E, K) and other essential nutrients due to malabsorption.
- Gastrointestinal Distress: Symptoms such as diarrhea, flatulence, and abdominal cramping may occur due to impaired digestion.

Diagnosis and Treatment

Diagnosing EPI typically involves a combination of clinical evaluation, laboratory tests, and imaging studies. Blood tests may be conducted to assess levels of pancreatic enzymes, while stool tests can detect fat malabsorption. Imaging techniques such as ultrasound, CT scan, or MRI may be used to visualize the pancreas and assess its structure and function.

Treatment for EPI aims to alleviate symptoms, improve nutritional status, and enhance quality of life. Central to EPI management is enzyme replacement therapy (ERT), which involves oral supplementation of pancreatic enzymes with meals to aid in digestion and nutrient absorption. Additionally, dietary modifications, nutritional counseling, and lifestyle interventions may be recommended to optimize digestive health and overall well-being.

CHAPTER 3

BASICS OF THE EPI DIET

The EPI (Exocrine Pancreatic Insufficiency) Diet is a specialized dietary approach designed to support individuals with EPI in managing their condition effectively. By focusing on optimizing nutrient absorption while minimizing digestive discomfort, the EPI Diet aims to improve overall health and quality of life for those affected by this gastrointestinal disorder.

Key Principles of the EPI Diet

Enzyme Replacement Therapy (ERT): Central to the EPI Diet is the use of enzyme replacement therapy. Since individuals with EPI lack sufficient pancreatic enzymes necessary for proper digestion, supplemental enzymes are taken with meals to aid in the breakdown of fats, proteins, and carbohydrates. These enzyme supplements help compensate for the pancreas's reduced enzyme production, facilitating better nutrient absorption and reducing symptoms such as steatorrhea (excess fat in the stool).

Balanced Nutrition: The EPI Diet emphasizes the importance of balanced nutrition to ensure adequate intake of essential nutrients. Meals should contain a combination of macronutrients, including carbohydrates, proteins, and fats, as well as micronutrients such as vitamins and minerals. By consuming a well-balanced diet, individuals with EPI can meet their nutritional needs and support overall health.

High-Calorie, High-Protein Foods: Due to the risk of unintentional weight loss and malnutrition associated with EPI, the diet often includes high-calorie, high-protein foods to help maintain or gain weight. Lean meats, poultry, fish, eggs, dairy products, legumes, and nuts are valuable sources of protein, while healthy fats from sources like avocados, olive oil, and nuts can provide additional calories and essential fatty acids.

Easily Digestible Foods: Given the impaired digestive function in EPI, it's essential to choose foods that are easy to digest and well-tolerated. This may involve cooking methods such as steaming, baking, or grilling to make foods more digestible. Avoiding high-fat, greasy, or heavily processed foods can help minimize digestive discomfort and improve overall digestion.

Frequent, Smaller Meals: Instead of consuming large meals infrequently, individuals with EPI may benefit from eating smaller, more frequent meals throughout the day. This eating pattern helps prevent overwhelming the digestive system and may reduce symptoms such as bloating, gas, and abdominal discomfort.

Hydration: Adequate hydration is essential for maintaining digestive health and preventing constipation, a common issue for individuals with EPI. Drinking plenty of water throughout the day can help promote regular bowel movements and support overall hydration status.

Dietary Considerations for EPI

In addition to following the key principles outlined above, individuals with EPI may benefit from specific dietary considerations, including:

Limiting High-Fat Foods: While healthy fats are an important part of the diet, individuals with EPI may need to limit their intake of high-fat foods, as these can be difficult to digest and may exacerbate symptoms of steatorrhea.

Monitoring Fiber Intake: Although fiber is essential for digestive health, consuming excessive amounts of fiber-rich foods may contribute to gastrointestinal discomfort for some individuals with EPI. It's essential to monitor fiber intake and adjust accordingly based on individual tolerance.

Avoiding Trigger Foods: Certain foods may trigger digestive symptoms in individuals with EPI. Keeping a food diary can help identify trigger foods and guide dietary modifications to minimize discomfort.

CHAPTER 4

CREATING YOUR EPI DIET MEAL PLAN

Calculating Caloric Needs

Determining your caloric needs is a crucial step in creating an effective EPI diet plan tailored to your individual requirements. Caloric needs vary based on factors such as age, gender, weight, height, activity level, and metabolic rate. By accurately calculating your caloric needs, you can ensure that your EPI diet provides adequate energy to support your daily activities while promoting optimal health and well-being.

Methods of Calculating Caloric Needs

Several methods can be used to estimate your caloric requirements:

Harris-Benedict Equation: This equation calculates basal metabolic rate (BMR), representing the number of calories your body needs at rest to maintain essential bodily functions. The formula varies based on gender and involves multiplying your weight, height, age, and gender-specific coefficients.

Total Energy Expenditure (TEE): TEE accounts for both BMR and physical activity level (PAL), providing a more comprehensive estimate of daily calorie needs. PAL factors in the calories burned through physical activity and ranges from sedentary to highly active.

Activity Multipliers: Activity multipliers can be applied to your BMR to estimate calorie needs based on your activity level. These multipliers typically range from 1.2 (sedentary) to 2.4 (very active), reflecting the additional calories expended through physical activity.

Example Calculation

Here's a simplified example of how to calculate caloric needs using the Harris-Benedict Equation and an activity multiplier:

Calculate Basal Metabolic Rate (BMR):

For males: BMR = 88.362 + (13.397 × weight in kg) + (4.799 × height in cm) - (5.677 × age in years)

For females: BMR = 447.593 + (9.247 × weight in kg) + (3.098 × height in cm) - (4.330 × age in years)

Apply Activity Multiplier:

Sedentary (little to no exercise): BMR × 1.2

Lightly active (light exercise/sports 1-3 days/week): BMR × 1.375

Moderately active (moderate exercise/sports 3-5 days/week): BMR × 1.55

Very active (hard exercise/sports 6-7 days a week): BMR × 1.725

Extra active (very hard exercise/sports & physical job or 2x training): BMR × 1.9

Adjust for Goals: Depending on your goals (e.g., weight maintenance, weight loss, or weight gain), you may need to adjust your calorie intake accordingly.

Importance of Accuracy

Accurately calculating your caloric needs lays the foundation for designing an EPI diet plan that meets your nutritional requirements while supporting your health goals. It's essential to be as precise as possible when estimating calorie needs to ensure that you're providing your body with the appropriate amount of energy for optimal functioning.

Determining Macronutrient Ratios

In addition to calculating total caloric needs, determining the appropriate macronutrient ratios is essential for creating a well-balanced EPI diet plan that supports optimal health and digestion. Macronutrients—carbohydrates, proteins, and fats—play distinct roles in providing energy, supporting cellular function, and maintaining overall nutritional status. By establishing the right balance of macronutrients, individuals with EPI can optimize nutrient absorption, manage symptoms, and promote overall well-being.

Understanding Macronutrients

Carbohydrates: Carbohydrates are the body's primary source of energy and play a crucial role in fueling cellular metabolism. Complex carbohydrates, found in whole grains, fruits, and vegetables, provide sustained energy and essential nutrients such as fiber, vitamins, and minerals.

Proteins: Proteins are essential for building and repairing tissues, synthesizing enzymes and hormones, and supporting immune function. High-quality protein sources, such as lean meats, poultry, fish, eggs, dairy products, legumes, and tofu, are rich in essential amino acids necessary for optimal health.

Fats: Dietary fats serve as a concentrated source of energy, provide essential fatty acids, and facilitate the absorption of fat-soluble vitamins (A, D, E, K). Healthy fats, including monounsaturated and polyunsaturated fats found in nuts, seeds, avocados, and fatty fish, support heart health and promote overall well-being.

Determining Macronutrient Ratios

The ideal macronutrient ratio for individuals with EPI may vary depending on factors such as metabolic rate, activity level, health goals, and tolerance to specific nutrients. However, a balanced approach that emphasizes quality sources of carbohydrates, proteins, and fats is generally recommended. Here are some guidelines for determining macronutrient ratios:

Carbohydrates: Aim to include a moderate amount of complex carbohydrates in your diet, focusing on whole grains, fruits, vegetables, and legumes. Complex carbohydrates provide sustained energy and essential nutrients while minimizing blood sugar fluctuations.

Proteins: Incorporate adequate protein into your diet to support muscle maintenance, tissue repair, and immune function. Choose lean protein sources such as poultry, fish, tofu, legumes, and low-fat dairy products, and distribute protein intake evenly throughout the day.

Fats: Include healthy fats in your diet from sources such as nuts, seeds, avocados, olive oil, and fatty fish. Aim to limit saturated and trans fats found in processed foods and fried items, as they can exacerbate digestive symptoms and contribute to inflammation.

Flexibility and Individualization

While establishing general macronutrient guidelines is helpful, it's essential to tailor your EPI diet plan to your individual needs, preferences, and tolerances. Some individuals may benefit from higher or lower carbohydrate or protein intake based on factors such as insulin sensitivity, metabolic rate, and digestive tolerance. Experimenting with different macronutrient ratios and adjusting your diet based on your body's response can help you find the optimal balance for managing EPI symptoms and promoting overall health.

Meal Planning Strategies

Effective meal planning is a cornerstone of the EPI diet, enabling individuals to manage their condition while enjoying a varied, nutritious diet. By implementing strategic meal planning strategies, individuals with EPI can ensure that their meals are well-balanced, easily digestible, and tailored to their specific nutritional needs. Here are some meal planning strategies to consider:

1. Focus on Nutrient-Dense Foods

Prioritize nutrient-dense foods that provide essential vitamins, minerals, and antioxidants to support overall health and well-being. Include a variety of colorful fruits and vegetables, whole grains, lean proteins, and healthy fats in your meals to ensure a broad spectrum of nutrients.

2. Opt for Easily Digestible Foods

Select foods that are gentle on the digestive system and easy to digest, reducing the risk of gastrointestinal discomfort and symptoms. Choose cooked or steamed vegetables over raw ones, opt for lean cuts of meat and poultry, and incorporate easily digestible grains such as rice and oats into your meals.

3. Small, Frequent Meals

Instead of three large meals, consider eating smaller, more frequent meals throughout the day to support digestion and nutrient absorption. Eating smaller portions at regular intervals can help prevent overloading the digestive system and minimize symptoms such as bloating and discomfort.

4. Incorporate Enzyme Replacement Therapy (ERT)

If prescribed by your healthcare provider, incorporate enzyme replacement therapy (ERT) into your meal planning routine. Take enzyme supplements with meals and snacks to aid in the digestion and absorption of nutrients, optimizing nutrient uptake and reducing digestive symptoms.

5. Balance Macronutrients

Ensure that your meals contain a balance of carbohydrates, proteins, and fats to provide sustained energy and support overall nutrition. Aim for a balanced macronutrient ratio that includes complex carbohydrates, lean proteins, and healthy fats in each meal to promote satiety and stability in blood sugar levels.

6. Plan Ahead and Prep Meals

Take time to plan your meals in advance and prepare ingredients ahead of time to streamline meal preparation and ensure consistency in your diet. Batch cooking, meal prepping, and storing meals in portion-sized containers can save time and effort during busy periods while maintaining adherence to your EPI diet plan.

7. Listen to Your Body

Pay attention to how your body responds to different foods and meal compositions, and adjust your meal plan accordingly. Keep a food diary to track symptoms, identify trigger foods, and pinpoint dietary patterns that work best for managing your EPI symptoms and promoting digestive health.

8. Stay Hydrated

Remember to stay hydrated by drinking an adequate amount of water throughout the day. Proper hydration supports digestion, nutrient absorption, and overall gastrointestinal health, helping to alleviate symptoms such as constipation and bloating commonly associated with EPI.

9. Seek Support and Guidance

Don't hesitate to seek support and guidance from healthcare professionals, registered dietitians, or support groups specializing in EPI management. They can provide personalized recommendations, practical tips, and emotional support to help you navigate the challenges of meal planning and optimize your dietary choices for managing EPI effectively.

CHAPTER 5

SAMPLE MEAL PLANS

Beginner's Week Meal Plan

Day 1:

- **Breakfast:** Scrambled eggs with spinach and tomatoes, served with whole-grain toast.
- **Mid-Morning Snack:** Greek yogurt with berries.
- **Lunch:** Grilled chicken breast salad with mixed greens, cucumber, bell peppers, and balsamic vinaigrette.
- **Afternoon Snack:** Sliced apples with almond butter.
- Dinner: Baked salmon with quinoa and steamed broccoli.

Day 2:

- **Breakfast:** Oatmeal topped with sliced bananas and a sprinkle of cinnamon.
- **Mid-Morning Snack:** Carrot sticks with hummus.
- **Lunch:** Turkey and avocado wrap with whole-grain tortilla, lettuce, and tomato.
- **Afternoon Snack:** Cottage cheese with pineapple chunks.

- **Dinner:** Stir-fried tofu with mixed vegetables and brown rice.

Day 3:

- **Breakfast:** Smoothie made with spinach, banana, almond milk, and protein powder.
- **Mid-Morning Snack:** Handful of almonds.
- **Lunch:** Quinoa salad with chickpeas, cherry tomatoes, cucumber, feta cheese, and lemon-tahini dressing.
- **Afternoon Snack:** Celery sticks with peanut butter.
- **Dinner:** Grilled shrimp skewers with roasted sweet potatoes and asparagus.

Day 4:

- **Breakfast:** Whole-grain toast topped with mashed avocado and poached eggs.
- **Mid-Morning Snack:** Greek yogurt with granola.
- **Lunch:** Lentil soup with a side of mixed green salad and whole-grain bread.
- **Afternoon Snack:** Sliced pear with cheese.
- **Dinner:** Baked chicken thighs with roasted Brussels sprouts and quinoa.

Day 5:

- **Breakfast:** Cottage cheese with sliced peaches and a drizzle of honey.
- **Mid-Morning Snack:** Baby carrots with tzatziki dip.
- **Lunch:** Spinach and feta omelet served with a side of mixed berries.
- **Afternoon Snack:** Trail mix with nuts and dried fruit.
- **Dinner:** Turkey meatballs with marinara sauce over zucchini noodles.

Day 6:

- **Breakfast:** Whole-grain pancakes topped with Greek yogurt and mixed berries.
- **Mid-Morning Snack:** Edamame beans.
- **Lunch:** Grilled vegetable and quinoa salad with a lemon-herb dressing.
- **Afternoon Snack:** Sliced cucumber with hummus.
- **Dinner:** Baked cod with roasted root vegetables and a side of barley.

Day 7:

- **Breakfast:** Scrambled tofu with sautéed spinach, bell peppers, and onions.
- **Mid-Morning Snack:** Apple slices with almond butter.

- **Lunch:** Chickpea salad with cherry tomatoes, cucumber, red onion, and a lemon-tahini dressing.
- **Afternoon Snack:** Cottage cheese with pineapple chunks.
- **Dinner:** Beef stir-fry with broccoli, snap peas, and brown rice.

Day 8:

- **Breakfast:** Whole-grain cereal with almond milk and sliced strawberries.
- **Mid-Morning Snack:** Celery sticks with cream cheese.
- **Lunch:** Grilled shrimp Caesar salad with romaine lettuce, cherry tomatoes, Parmesan cheese, and Caesar dressing.
- **Afternoon Snack:** Mixed nuts and dried fruit.
- **Dinner:** Baked turkey breast with sweet potato mash and steamed green beans.

Day 9:

- **Breakfast:** Banana protein smoothie made with almond milk, protein powder, spinach, and almond butter.
- **Mid-Morning Snack:** Rice cakes with avocado mash.

- **Lunch:** Quinoa and black bean stuffed bell peppers with a side of salsa and guacamole.
- **Afternoon Snack:** Sliced mango with cottage cheese.
- **Dinner:** Baked salmon with roasted cauliflower and quinoa.

Day 10:

- **Breakfast:** Whole-grain waffles with Greek yogurt and sliced peaches.
- **Mid-Morning Snack:** Cherry tomatoes with mozzarella cheese.
- **Lunch:** Lentil and vegetable soup with a side of whole-grain bread.
- **Afternoon Snack:** Apple slices with almond butter.
- **Dinner:** Chicken and vegetable stir-fry with brown rice.

Day 11:

- **Breakfast:** Scrambled eggs with sautéed spinach, mushrooms, and onions.
- **Mid-Morning Snack:** Baby carrots with hummus.
- **Lunch:** Tuna salad with mixed greens, cherry tomatoes, cucumber, and balsamic vinaigrette.

- **Afternoon Snack:** Cottage cheese with pineapple chunks.
- **Dinner:** Baked tofu with roasted Brussels sprouts and quinoa.

Day 12:

- **Breakfast:** Overnight oats with almond milk, chia seeds, and mixed berries.
- **Mid-Morning Snack:** Rice cakes with peanut butter.
- **Lunch:** Turkey and avocado wrap with whole-grain tortilla, lettuce, tomato, and mustard.
- **Afternoon Snack:** Greek yogurt with honey and walnuts.
- **Dinner:** Beef and vegetable kebabs with grilled zucchini and couscous.

Day 13:

- **Breakfast:** Whole-grain toast with mashed avocado and poached eggs.
- **Mid-Morning Snack:** Edamame beans.
- **Lunch:** Spinach and feta quiche with a side of mixed berries.
- **Afternoon Snack:** Sliced cucumber with tzatziki dip.
- **Dinner:** Baked cod with roasted sweet potatoes and steamed broccoli.

Day 14:

- **Breakfast:** Smoothie bowl made with mixed berries, banana, Greek yogurt, and granola.
- **Mid-Morning Snack:** Mixed nuts and dried fruit.
- **Lunch:** Chicken and vegetable curry with brown rice.
- **Afternoon Snack:** Carrot sticks with hummus.
- **Dinner:** Lentil and vegetable stew served with whole-grain bread.

Day 15:

- **Breakfast:** Whole-grain pancakes topped with Greek yogurt and mixed berries.
- **Mid-Morning Snack:** Apple slices with almond butter.
- **Lunch:** Quinoa salad with roasted vegetables, chickpeas, and a lemon-tahini dressing.
- **Afternoon Snack:** Cottage cheese with sliced peaches.
- **Dinner:** Baked chicken thighs with sweet potato wedges and steamed green beans.

Day 16:

- **Breakfast:** Scrambled eggs with diced bell peppers, onions, and tomatoes, served with whole-grain toast.
- **Mid-Morning Snack:** Baby carrots with hummus.
- **Lunch:** Grilled vegetable and feta cheese wrap with whole-grain tortilla.
- **Afternoon Snack:** Greek yogurt with honey and walnuts.
- **Dinner:** Baked salmon with quinoa pilaf and sautéed spinach.

Day 17:

- **Breakfast:** Smoothie made with spinach, banana, almond milk, and protein powder.
- **Mid-Morning Snack:** Rice cakes with avocado mash and cherry tomatoes.
- **Lunch:** Turkey and avocado salad with mixed greens, cucumber, and balsamic vinaigrette.
- **Afternoon Snack:** Sliced pear with cheese.
- **Dinner:** Beef and vegetable stir-fry with brown rice.

Day 18:

- **Breakfast:** Overnight oats with almond milk, chia seeds, and sliced strawberries.
- **Mid-Morning Snack:** Mixed nuts and dried fruit.

- **Lunch:** Lentil soup with a side of whole-grain bread and mixed green salad.
- **Afternoon Snack:** Greek yogurt with granola and sliced banana.
- **Dinner:** Baked tofu with roasted Brussels sprouts and quinoa.

Day 19:

- **Breakfast:** Whole-grain toast with mashed avocado and poached eggs.
- **Mid-Morning Snack:** Carrot sticks with hummus.
- **Lunch:** Grilled chicken Caesar salad with romaine lettuce, cherry tomatoes, Parmesan cheese, and Caesar dressing.
- **Afternoon Snack:** Cottage cheese with pineapple chunks.
- **Dinner:** Baked cod with roasted sweet potatoes and steamed broccoli.

Day 20:

- **Breakfast:** Greek yogurt parfait with layers of granola, mixed berries, and honey.
- **Mid-Morning Snack:** Celery sticks with cream cheese and sunflower seeds.

- **Lunch:** Chickpea and vegetable curry with brown rice.
- **Afternoon Snack:** Sliced apple with almond butter.
- **Dinner:** Turkey meatballs with marinara sauce over zucchini noodles.

Day 21:

- **Breakfast:** Whole-grain waffles with sliced banana and a drizzle of maple syrup.
- **Mid-Morning Snack:** Edamame beans.
- **Lunch:** Quinoa and black bean salad with diced tomatoes, corn, and avocado.
- **Afternoon Snack:** Mixed nuts and dried fruit.
- **Dinner:** Beef and vegetable kebabs with grilled bell peppers, onions, and quinoa.

Intermediate Week Meal Plan

Day 1:

- **Breakfast:** Scrambled eggs with sautéed spinach, bell peppers, and onions, served with whole-grain toast.
- **Mid-Morning Snack:** Greek yogurt with sliced strawberries and a drizzle of honey.

- **Lunch:** Grilled chicken breast salad with mixed greens, cherry tomatoes, cucumber, avocado, and balsamic vinaigrette.
- **Afternoon Snack:** Carrot sticks with hummus.
- **Dinner:** Baked salmon with quinoa pilaf and roasted asparagus.

Day 2:

- **Breakfast:** Oatmeal topped with sliced bananas, chopped walnuts, and a sprinkle of cinnamon.
- **Mid-Morning Snack:** Apple slices with almond butter.
- **Lunch:** Turkey and avocado wrap with whole-grain tortilla, lettuce, tomato, and mustard.
- **Afternoon Snack:** Greek yogurt with granola and mixed berries.
- **Dinner:** Lentil and vegetable stew served with a side of whole-grain bread.

Day 3:

- **Breakfast:** Whole-grain pancakes topped with Greek yogurt, mixed berries, and a drizzle of maple syrup.
- **Mid-Morning Snack:** Cottage cheese with pineapple chunks.

- **Lunch:** Quinoa salad with chickpeas, cherry tomatoes, cucumber, feta cheese, and lemon-tahini dressing.
- **Afternoon Snack:** Rice cakes with avocado mash and cherry tomatoes.
- **Dinner:** Baked chicken thighs with roasted sweet potatoes and steamed green beans.

Day 4:

- **Breakfast:** Smoothie made with spinach, banana, almond milk, protein powder, and almond butter.
- **Mid-Morning Snack:** Mixed nuts and dried fruit.
- **Lunch:** Tuna salad with mixed greens, cherry tomatoes, cucumber, hard-boiled eggs, and balsamic vinaigrette.
- **Afternoon Snack:** Celery sticks with cream cheese and sunflower seeds.
- **Dinner:** Grilled shrimp skewers with quinoa tabbouleh and grilled zucchini.

Day 5:

- **Breakfast:** Whole-grain toast with mashed avocado, poached eggs, and a sprinkle of red pepper flakes.
- **Mid-Morning Snack:** Sliced pear with cheese.

- **Lunch:** Spinach and feta quiche with a side of mixed green salad and whole-grain bread.
- **Afternoon Snack:** Greek yogurt with honey and sliced almonds.
- **Dinner:** Baked cod with roasted Brussels sprouts and brown rice.

Day 6:

- **Breakfast:** Scrambled tofu with sautéed mushrooms, onions, and cherry tomatoes, served with whole-grain toast.
- **Mid-Morning Snack:** Carrot sticks with hummus.
- **Lunch:** Chicken and vegetable stir-fry with brown rice.
- **Afternoon Snack:** Cottage cheese with sliced peaches.
- **Dinner:** Beef and broccoli stir-fry with quinoa.

Day 7:

- **Breakfast:** Overnight oats with almond milk, chia seeds, sliced almonds, and mixed berries.
- **Mid-Morning Snack:** Baby carrots with tzatziki dip.
- **Lunch:** Grilled vegetable and quinoa salad with a lemon-herb dressing.

- **Afternoon Snack:** Rice cakes with almond butter and sliced banana.
- **Dinner:** Turkey meatballs with marinara sauce over zucchini noodles.

Day 8:

- **Breakfast:** Scrambled eggs with sautéed spinach, mushrooms, and onions, served with whole-grain toast.
- **Mid-Morning Snack:** Greek yogurt with mixed berries and a drizzle of honey.
- **Lunch:** Grilled chicken breast salad with mixed greens, cherry tomatoes, cucumber, avocado, and balsamic vinaigrette.
- **Afternoon Snack:** Carrot sticks with hummus.
- **Dinner:** Baked salmon with quinoa pilaf and roasted asparagus.

Day 9:

- **Breakfast:** Oatmeal topped with sliced bananas, chopped walnuts, and a sprinkle of cinnamon.
- **Mid-Morning Snack:** Cottage cheese with pineapple chunks.
- **Lunch:** Lentil and vegetable soup with a side of whole-grain bread.

- **Afternoon Snack:** Rice cakes with almond butter and sliced strawberries.
- **Dinner:** Turkey and vegetable stir-fry with brown rice.

Day 10:

- **Breakfast:** Whole-grain toast with mashed avocado and poached eggs, sprinkled with black sesame seeds.
- **Mid-Morning Snack:** Mixed nuts and dried fruit.
- **Lunch:** Tuna salad with mixed greens, cherry tomatoes, cucumber, olives, and lemon-tahini dressing.
- **Afternoon Snack:** Sliced apple with peanut butter.
- Dinner: Baked tofu with steamed broccoli and quinoa.

Day 11:

- **Breakfast:** Smoothie made with spinach, banana, almond milk, protein powder, and a spoonful of almond butter.
- **Mid-Morning Snack:** Baby carrots with tzatziki dip.
- **Lunch:** Chickpea and avocado wrap with whole-grain tortilla, lettuce, tomato, and hummus.

- **Afternoon Snack:** Greek yogurt with granola and sliced peaches.
- **Dinner:** Grilled shrimp skewers with roasted sweet potatoes and green beans.

Day 12:

- **Breakfast:** Whole-grain pancakes topped with Greek yogurt and mixed berries.
- **Mid-Morning Snack:** Sliced cucumber with cream cheese and dill.
- **Lunch:** Quinoa and black bean salad with diced bell peppers, corn, avocado, and lime-cilantro dressing.
- **Afternoon Snack:** Cottage cheese with sliced pears and a sprinkle of cinnamon.
- **Dinner:** Beef and vegetable curry with brown rice.

Day 13:

- **Breakfast:** Scrambled eggs with diced bell peppers, onions, and tomatoes, served with whole-grain toast.
- **Mid-Morning Snack:** Rice cakes with avocado mash and cherry tomatoes.
- **Lunch:** Grilled vegetable and feta cheese wrap with whole-grain tortilla and tzatziki sauce.

- **Afternoon Snack:** Mixed nuts and dried cranberries.
- **Dinner:** Baked cod with roasted Brussels sprouts and quinoa.

Day 14:

- **Breakfast:** Overnight oats with almond milk, chia seeds, sliced strawberries, and a drizzle of maple syrup.
- **Mid-Morning Snack:** Greek yogurt with honey and chopped almonds.
- **Lunch:** Spinach and feta quiche with a side salad of mixed greens, cherry tomatoes, and balsamic vinaigrette.
- **Afternoon Snack:** Apple slices with almond butter.
- **Dinner:** Turkey meatballs with marinara sauce over zucchini noodles.
- Feel free to adjust portion sizes and ingredients based on your individual preferences and dietary needs. Enjoy your meals!

Day 15:

- **Breakfast:** Whole-grain toast topped with mashed avocado, smoked salmon, and a sprinkle of black pepper.

- **Mid-Morning Snack:** Greek yogurt with mixed berries and a drizzle of honey.
- **Lunch:** Quinoa salad with roasted vegetables (such as bell peppers, zucchini, and eggplant), chickpeas, and a lemon-tahini dressing.
- **Afternoon Snack:** Carrot sticks with hummus.
- **Dinner:** Grilled chicken breast with quinoa pilaf and steamed green beans.

Day 16:

- **Breakfast:** Scrambled eggs with diced tomatoes, spinach, and feta cheese, served with whole-grain toast.
- **Mid-Morning Snack:** Cottage cheese with sliced peaches.
- **Lunch:** Lentil soup with a side of mixed green salad and whole-grain bread.
- **Afternoon Snack:** Rice cakes with almond butter and banana slices.
- **Dinner:** Baked salmon with roasted sweet potatoes and sautéed spinach.

Day 17:

- **Breakfast:** Oatmeal topped with sliced bananas, chopped walnuts, and a drizzle of maple syrup.

- **Mid-Morning Snack:** Mixed nuts and dried fruit.
- **Lunch:** Tuna salad with mixed greens, cherry tomatoes, cucumber, olives, and lemon-tahini dressing.
- **Afternoon Snack:** Sliced apple with peanut butter.
- **Dinner:** Beef and vegetable stir-fry with brown rice.

Day 18:

- **Breakfast:** Smoothie made with spinach, banana, almond milk, protein powder, and a spoonful of almond butter.
- **Mid-Morning Snack:** Baby carrots with hummus.
- **Lunch:** Chickpea and avocado wrap with whole-grain tortilla, lettuce, tomato, and hummus.
- **Afternoon Snack:** Greek yogurt with granola and sliced strawberries.
- **Dinner:** Grilled shrimp skewers with quinoa pilaf and steamed broccoli.

Day 19:

- **Breakfast:** Whole-grain pancakes topped with Greek yogurt and mixed berries.
- **Mid-Morning Snack:** Sliced cucumber with cream cheese and dill.

- **Lunch:** Quinoa and black bean salad with diced bell peppers, corn, avocado, and lime-cilantro dressing.
- **Afternoon Snack:** Cottage cheese with sliced pears and a sprinkle of cinnamon.
- **Dinner:** Baked tofu with stir-fried vegetables (such as bell peppers, snap peas, and carrots) and brown rice.

Day 20:

- **Breakfast:** Scrambled eggs with sautéed mushrooms, onions, and spinach, served with whole-grain toast.
- **Mid-Morning Snack:** Rice cakes with avocado mash and cherry tomatoes.
- **Lunch:** Grilled vegetable and feta cheese wrap with whole-grain tortilla and tzatziki sauce.
- **Afternoon Snack:** Mixed nuts and dried cranberries.
- **Dinner:** Baked cod with roasted Brussels sprouts and quinoa.

Day 21:

- **Breakfast:** Overnight oats with almond milk, chia seeds, sliced strawberries, and a drizzle of honey.

- **Mid-Morning Snack:** Greek yogurt with honey and chopped almonds.
- **Lunch:** Spinach and feta quiche with a side salad of mixed greens, cherry tomatoes, and balsamic vinaigrette.
- **Afternoon Snack:** Apple slices with almond butter.
- **Dinner:** Turkey meatballs with marinara sauce over zucchini noodles.

Advanced Week Meal Plan

Day 1:

- **Breakfast:** Avocado toast on whole-grain bread topped with poached eggs and a sprinkle of black pepper.
- **Mid-Morning Snack:** Greek yogurt parfait with layers of mixed berries and granola.
- **Lunch:** Grilled chicken breast with quinoa and roasted vegetables (bell peppers, zucchini, and eggplant).
- **Afternoon Snack:** Sliced apples with almond butter.
- **Dinner:** Baked salmon with lemon-dill sauce, served with steamed asparagus and wild rice.
- **Day 2:**

- **Breakfast:** Smoothie bowl made with spinach, banana, almond milk, protein powder, and topped with sliced strawberries and chia seeds.
- **Mid-Morning Snack:** Cottage cheese with pineapple chunks and a drizzle of honey.
- **Lunch:** Lentil and vegetable stir-fry with tofu, broccoli, carrots, and snap peas, served over brown rice.
- **Afternoon Snack:** Mixed nuts and dried fruit.
- **Dinner:** Turkey meatballs in marinara sauce over whole-grain spaghetti, served with a side of mixed green salad.

Day 3:

- **Breakfast:** Whole-grain pancakes topped with Greek yogurt, mixed berries, and a sprinkle of crushed nuts.
- **Mid-Morning Snack:** Rice cakes with avocado mash and cherry tomatoes.
- **Lunch:** Grilled shrimp Caesar salad with romaine lettuce, cherry tomatoes, Parmesan cheese, and Caesar dressing.
- **Afternoon Snack:** Carrot sticks with hummus.
- **Dinner:** Beef and vegetable curry with cauliflower rice and steamed green beans.

Day 4:

- **Breakfast:** Veggie-packed omelet with spinach, bell peppers, onions, tomatoes, and feta cheese, served with whole-grain toast.
- **Mid-Morning Snack:** Greek yogurt with sliced peaches and a drizzle of maple syrup.
- **Lunch:** Quinoa and black bean salad with diced avocado, corn, red onion, and cilantro-lime dressing.
- **Afternoon Snack:** Sliced cucumbers with tzatziki dip.
- **Dinner:** Baked cod with mango salsa, served with quinoa pilaf and roasted Brussels sprouts.

Day 5:

- **Breakfast:** Overnight oats with almond milk, chia seeds, sliced bananas, and a dollop of almond butter.
- **Mid-Morning Snack:** Mixed berries with cottage cheese and a sprinkle of cinnamon.
- **Lunch:** Turkey and avocado wrap with whole-grain tortilla, lettuce, tomato, and mustard.
- **Afternoon Snack:** Edamame beans.

- **Dinner:** Grilled vegetable and chickpea salad with mixed greens, cherry tomatoes, cucumber, and lemon-tahini dressing.

Day 6:

- **Breakfast:** Whole-grain waffles topped with Greek yogurt, sliced strawberries, and a drizzle of honey.
- **Mid-Morning Snack:** Rice cakes with almond butter and banana slices.
- **Lunch:** Spinach and feta quiche with a side of mixed green salad and balsamic vinaigrette.
- **Afternoon Snack:** Celery sticks with cream cheese and sunflower seeds.
- **Dinner:** Baked tofu with stir-fried bok choy, bell peppers, and brown rice.

Day 7:

- **Breakfast:** Scrambled eggs with smoked salmon, diced avocado, and whole-grain toast.
- **Mid-Morning Snack:** Greek yogurt with granola and mixed berries.
- **Lunch:** Chicken and vegetable curry with quinoa and steamed broccoli.
- **Afternoon Snack:** Sliced pear with cheese.

- **Dinner:** Beef stir-fry with snap peas, carrots, and bell peppers, served with cauliflower rice.

Day 8:

- **Breakfast:** Quinoa breakfast bowl with scrambled eggs, sautéed spinach, cherry tomatoes, and avocado slices.
- **Mid-Morning Snack:** Greek yogurt with sliced peaches and a drizzle of honey.
- **Lunch:** Grilled chicken salad with mixed greens, strawberries, feta cheese, and balsamic vinaigrette.
- **Afternoon Snack:** Carrot sticks with hummus.
- **Dinner:** Baked salmon with roasted sweet potatoes and green beans.

Day 9:

- **Breakfast:** Whole-grain toast topped with mashed avocado, poached eggs, and a sprinkle of red pepper flakes.
- **Mid-Morning Snack:** Cottage cheese with pineapple chunks and a sprinkle of cinnamon.
- **Lunch:** Lentil and vegetable soup with a side of whole-grain bread.
- **Afternoon Snack:** Rice cakes with almond butter and banana slices.

- **Dinner:** Turkey and vegetable stir-fry with brown rice.

Day 10:

- **Breakfast:** Smoothie made with spinach, banana, almond milk, protein powder, and a spoonful of almond butter.
- **Mid-Morning Snack:** Mixed nuts and dried fruit.
- **Lunch:** Tuna salad with mixed greens, cherry tomatoes, cucumber, olives, and lemon-tahini dressing.
- **Afternoon Snack:** Sliced apple with peanut butter.
- **Dinner:** Baked tofu with quinoa and roasted vegetables (bell peppers, zucchini, and carrots).

Day 11:

- **Breakfast:** Greek yogurt parfait with layers of granola, mixed berries, and sliced almonds.
- **Mid-Morning Snack:** Baby carrots with tzatziki dip.
- **Lunch:** Grilled shrimp Caesar salad with romaine lettuce, cherry tomatoes, Parmesan cheese, and Caesar dressing.
- **Afternoon Snack:** Mixed berries with cottage cheese and a sprinkle of cinnamon.

- **Dinner:** Beef and vegetable curry with cauliflower rice and steamed broccoli.

Day 12:

- **Breakfast:** Veggie-packed omelet with spinach, mushrooms, onions, bell peppers, and feta cheese.
- **Mid-Morning Snack:** Greek yogurt with sliced mango and a drizzle of honey.
- **Lunch:** Quinoa and black bean salad with diced avocado, corn, red onion, and lime-cilantro dressing.
- **Afternoon Snack:** Sliced cucumber with hummus.
- **Dinner:** Baked cod with mango salsa, served with quinoa pilaf and roasted Brussels sprouts.

Day 13:

- **Breakfast:** Overnight oats with almond milk, chia seeds, sliced bananas, and a dollop of almond butter.
- **Mid-Morning Snack:** Rice cakes with avocado mash and cherry tomatoes.
- **Lunch:** Turkey and avocado wrap with whole-grain tortilla, lettuce, tomato, and mustard.
- **Afternoon Snack:** Edamame beans.

- **Dinner:** Grilled vegetable and chickpea salad with mixed greens, cherry tomatoes, cucumber, and lemon-tahini dressing.

Day 14:

- **Breakfast:** Whole-grain waffles topped with Greek yogurt, mixed berries, and a drizzle of maple syrup.
- **Mid-Morning Snack:** Cottage cheese with sliced peaches and a sprinkle of granola.
- **Lunch:** Spinach and feta quiche with a side of mixed green salad and balsamic vinaigrette.
- **Afternoon Snack:** Celery sticks with cream cheese and sunflower seeds.
- **Dinner:** Baked tofu with stir-fried bok choy, bell peppers, and brown rice.

Day 15:

- **Breakfast:** Avocado and spinach smoothie made with almond milk, banana, spinach, avocado, and a scoop of protein powder.
- **Mid-Morning Snack:** Cottage cheese with sliced peaches and a sprinkle of cinnamon.
- **Lunch:** Grilled chicken Caesar salad with romaine lettuce, cherry tomatoes, Parmesan cheese, whole-grain croutons, and Caesar dressing.

- **Afternoon Snack:** Greek yogurt with mixed berries and a drizzle of honey.
- **Dinner:** Baked salmon with roasted sweet potatoes, steamed broccoli, and quinoa.

Day 16:

- **Breakfast:** Whole-grain toast topped with scrambled eggs, sautéed spinach, cherry tomatoes, and feta cheese.
- **Mid-Morning Snack:** Sliced cucumber with hummus.
- **Lunch:** Lentil soup with a side of mixed green salad and whole-grain bread.
- **Afternoon Snack:** Apple slices with almond butter.
- **Dinner:** Turkey and vegetable stir-fry with brown rice noodles.

Day 17:

- **Breakfast:** Veggie-packed breakfast burrito with scrambled eggs, black beans, bell peppers, onions, and salsa wrapped in a whole-grain tortilla.
- **Mid-Morning** Snack: Greek yogurt with granola and sliced strawberries.

- **Lunch:** Quinoa and black bean stuffed bell peppers topped with melted cheese and served with a side of guacamole.
- **Afternoon Snack:** Mixed nuts and dried fruit.
- **Dinner:** Baked cod with lemon-garlic butter sauce, roasted Brussels sprouts, and wild rice.

Day 18:

- **Breakfast:** Spinach and mushroom omelet with diced tomatoes and shredded mozzarella cheese, served with whole-grain toast.
- **Mid-Morning Snack:** Carrot sticks with tzatziki dip.
- **Lunch:** Grilled vegetable and quinoa salad with mixed greens, cherry tomatoes, cucumber, feta cheese, and balsamic vinaigrette.
- **Afternoon Snack:** Cottage cheese with pineapple chunks.
- **Dinner:** Beef and broccoli stir-fry with brown rice.

Day 19:

- **Breakfast:** Banana and almond butter smoothie made with almond milk, banana, almond butter, and a scoop of protein powder.
- **Mid-Morning Snack:** Rice cakes with avocado mash and cherry tomatoes.

- **Lunch:** Turkey and avocado wrap with whole-grain tortilla, lettuce, tomato, and hummus.
- **Afternoon Snack:** Mixed berries with cottage cheese and a drizzle of honey.
- **Dinner:** Grilled shrimp skewers with quinoa tabbouleh and roasted vegetables.

Day 20:

- **Breakfast:** Whole-grain pancakes topped with Greek yogurt, mixed berries, and a drizzle of maple syrup.
- **Mid-Morning Snack:** Edamame beans.
- **Lunch:** Chicken and vegetable curry with coconut milk, served with brown rice.
- **Afternoon Snack:** Sliced apple with peanut butter.
- **Dinner:** Baked tofu with stir-fried vegetables and soba noodles.

Day 21:

- **Breakfast:** Scrambled eggs with diced avocado, cherry tomatoes, and feta cheese, served with whole-grain toast.
- **Mid-Morning Snack:** Greek yogurt with granola and sliced peaches.

- **Lunch:** Quinoa salad with roasted vegetables, chickpeas, feta cheese, and lemon-tahini dressing.
- **Afternoon Snack:** Carrot sticks with hummus.
- **Dinner:** Baked salmon with roasted Brussels sprouts, sweet potato mash, and a side of mixed green salad.

CHAPTER 6

RECIPES FOR EPI DIET MEALS

Breakfast Recipes

1. Scrambled Tofu Breakfast Bowl

Ingredients:

- 1 tablespoon olive oil
- 1 block (14 oz) firm tofu, drained and crumbled
- 1 bell pepper, diced
- 1 small onion, diced
- 2 cloves garlic, minced
- 1 teaspoon ground turmeric
- 1/2 teaspoon ground cumin
- Salt and pepper to taste
- 2 cups fresh spinach leaves
- 1 avocado, sliced
- 1 tablespoon nutritional yeast (optional)
- Fresh cilantro or parsley for garnish

Directions:

- Heat olive oil in a large skillet over medium heat. Add diced onion, bell pepper, and minced garlic. Cook until softened, about 5 minutes.

- Add crumbled tofu to the skillet, along with turmeric, cumin, salt, and pepper. Cook for 5-7 minutes, stirring occasionally, until tofu is heated through and evenly coated with spices.
- Add fresh spinach leaves to the skillet and cook until wilted, about 2 minutes.
- Serve the scrambled tofu mixture in bowls, topped with sliced avocado and a sprinkle of nutritional yeast if desired. Garnish with fresh cilantro or parsley.

Nutrition Facts (per serving):

- Calories: 256
- Fat: 16.8g
- Saturated Fat: 2.3g
- Cholesterol: 0mg
- Sodium: 176mg
- Carbohydrate: 15.4g
- Protein: 14.2g
- Fiber: 8.7g
- Calcium: 143mg
- Iron: 3.7mg
- Potassium: 775mg

Prep Time: 15 mins

Total Time: 20 mins

Servings: 2

2. Vegetable Egg Muffins

Ingredients:

- 6 large eggs
- 1/2 cup diced bell peppers (any color)
- 1/2 cup diced mushrooms
- 1/4 cup diced onions
- 1/4 cup chopped spinach
- 1/4 cup diced tomatoes
- 1/4 cup shredded cheese (optional)
- Salt and pepper to taste
- Cooking spray

Directions:

- Preheat your oven to 350°F (175°C). Grease a muffin tin with cooking spray.
- In a mixing bowl, whisk together the eggs until well beaten. Season with salt and pepper.
- Divide the diced vegetables evenly among the muffin cups.
- Pour the beaten eggs over the vegetables, filling each muffin cup about 3/4 full.

- Sprinkle shredded cheese on top of each muffin, if using.
- Bake in the preheated oven for 20-25 minutes, or until the egg muffins are set and lightly golden on top.
- Remove from the oven and let cool for a few minutes before serving.

Nutrition Facts (per serving, 2 egg muffins):

- Calories: 165
- Fat: 10.9g
- Saturated Fat: 3.8g
- Cholesterol: 341mg
- Sodium: 194mg
- Carbohydrate: 3.4g
- Protein: 13.6g
- Fiber: 0.9g
- Calcium: 88mg
- Iron: 1.6mg
- Potassium: 217mg

Prep Time: 10 mins

Total Time: 35 mins

Servings: 3

3. Greek Yogurt Parfait

Ingredients:

- 1 cup Greek yogurt (unsweetened)
- 1/2 cup mixed berries (such as strawberries, blueberries, and raspberries)
- 1/4 cup granola
- 1 tablespoon honey (optional)
- Fresh mint leaves for garnish (optional)

Directions:

- In a serving glass or bowl, layer half of the Greek yogurt.
- Add half of the mixed berries on top of the yogurt layer.
- Sprinkle half of the granola over the berries.
- Repeat the layers with the remaining yogurt, berries, and granola.
- Drizzle honey over the top, if desired, for added sweetness.
- Garnish with fresh mint leaves for a pop of color and freshness.
- Serve immediately or refrigerate until ready to eat.

Nutrition Facts (per serving):

- Calories: 265
- Fat: 5.5g
- Saturated Fat: 1.2g
- Cholesterol: 10mg
- Sodium: 52mg
- Carbohydrate: 35.4g
- Protein: 17.8g
- Fiber: 4.5g
- Calcium: 223mg
- Iron: 1.3mg
- Potassium: 404mg

Prep Time: 5 mins

Total Time: 5 mins

Servings: 1

4. Avocado and Egg Breakfast Sandwich

Ingredients:

- 1 ripe avocado
- 2 eggs
- 2 whole-grain English muffins, split and toasted
- Salt and pepper to taste
- Optional toppings: sliced tomato, baby spinach leaves, cooked bacon or turkey bacon

Directions:

- Slice the avocado in half, remove the pit, and scoop the flesh into a bowl. Mash the avocado with a fork until smooth.
- In a non-stick skillet, fry the eggs to your desired doneness (fried, scrambled, or poached). Season with salt and pepper.
- Spread the mashed avocado evenly onto each toasted English muffin half.
- Place a cooked egg on top of the avocado spread on each English muffin.
- Add any desired toppings such as sliced tomato, baby spinach leaves, or cooked bacon.
- Place the other half of the English muffin on top to form a sandwich.
- Serve immediately and enjoy!

Nutrition Facts (per serving):

- Calories: 340
- Fat: 18g
- Saturated Fat: 4g
- Cholesterol: 195mg
- Sodium: 355mg
- Carbohydrate: 30g

- Protein: 15g
- Fiber: 7g
- Calcium: 80mg
- Iron: 2mg
- Potassium: 565mg

Prep Time: 10 mins

Total Time: 10 mins

Servings: 2

5. Banana and Peanut Butter Overnight Oats

Ingredients:

- 1/2 cup rolled oats
- 1/2 cup unsweetened almond milk (or any milk of choice)
- 1 ripe banana, mashed
- 2 tablespoons natural peanut butter
- 1 tablespoon chia seeds (optional)
- 1 teaspoon honey or maple syrup (optional)
- Sliced banana and a sprinkle of cinnamon for garnish (optional)

Directions:

- In a jar or container, combine rolled oats, almond milk, mashed banana, peanut butter, and chia seeds (if using). Stir well to combine all ingredients.
- If desired, sweeten with honey or maple syrup to taste.
- Cover the jar/container and refrigerate overnight or for at least 4 hours to allow the oats to soften and absorb the liquid.
- Before serving, give the oats a good stir. If the mixture is too thick, you can add a splash of almond milk to reach your desired consistency.
- Top with sliced banana and a sprinkle of cinnamon, if desired, before serving.

Nutrition Facts (per serving):

- Calories: 389
- Fat: 17g
- Saturated Fat: 3g
- Cholesterol: 0mg
- Sodium: 136mg
- Carbohydrate: 48g
- Protein: 12g
- Fiber: 8g
- Calcium: 115mg
- Iron: 2mg

- Potassium: 538mg

Prep Time: 5 mins

Total Time: Overnight

Servings: 1

Lunch Recipes

1. Quinoa and Black Bean Salad

Ingredients:

- 1 cup quinoa
- 1 can (15 oz) black beans, drained and rinsed
- 1 cup cherry tomatoes, halved
- 1/2 cup diced red bell pepper
- 1/4 cup chopped fresh cilantro
- 1/4 cup diced red onion
- 2 tablespoons lime juice
- 2 tablespoons olive oil
- 1 teaspoon ground cumin
- Salt and pepper to taste
- Optional toppings: avocado slices, crumbled feta cheese

Directions:

- Rinse quinoa under cold water. In a saucepan, combine quinoa with 2 cups of water. Bring to a boil, then reduce heat to low, cover, and simmer for 15-20 minutes, or until quinoa is cooked and water is absorbed. Remove from heat and let it cool.
- In a large mixing bowl, combine cooked quinoa, black beans, cherry tomatoes, red bell pepper, cilantro, and red onion.
- In a small bowl, whisk together lime juice, olive oil, cumin, salt, and pepper to make the dressing.
- Pour the dressing over the quinoa mixture and toss until well combined.
- Serve the salad chilled or at room temperature, garnished with avocado slices and crumbled feta cheese if desired.

Nutrition Facts (per serving):

- Calories: 307
- Fat: 9g
- Saturated Fat: 1g
- Cholesterol: 0mg
- Sodium: 187mg
- Carbohydrate: 48g
- Protein: 11g
- Fiber: 9g

- Calcium: 47mg
- Iron: 3mg
- Potassium: 646mg

Prep Time: 10 mins

Total Time: 30 mins

Servings: 4

2. Grilled Chicken Caesar Salad

Ingredients:

- 2 boneless, skinless chicken breasts
- 1 tablespoon olive oil
- Salt and pepper to taste
- 1 head romaine lettuce, washed and chopped
- 1/4 cup grated Parmesan cheese
- 1/2 cup croutons
- Caesar dressing (store-bought or homemade)

Directions:

- Preheat the grill to medium-high heat.
- Brush the chicken breasts with olive oil and season with salt and pepper.
- Grill the chicken breasts for 6-8 minutes per side, or until cooked through and no longer pink in the center.

Remove from the grill and let them rest for a few minutes before slicing.
- In a large salad bowl, combine the chopped romaine lettuce, grated Parmesan cheese, and croutons.
- Add the sliced grilled chicken to the salad bowl.
- Drizzle Caesar dressing over the salad and toss until everything is evenly coated.
- Serve the Grilled Chicken Caesar Salad immediately, garnished with additional Parmesan cheese and croutons if desired.

Nutrition Facts (per serving):

- Calories: 320
- Fat: 14g
- Saturated Fat: 4g
- Cholesterol: 90mg
- Sodium: 560mg
- Carbohydrate: 10g
- Protein: 38g
- Fiber: 3g
- Calcium: 100mg
- Iron: 2mg
- Potassium: 650mg

Prep Time: 10 mins

Total Time: 20 mins

Servings: 2

3. Mediterranean Chickpea Salad

Ingredients:

- 1 can (15 oz) chickpeas, drained and rinsed
- 1 cup cherry tomatoes, halved
- 1/2 cucumber, diced
- 1/4 cup diced red onion
- 1/4 cup chopped fresh parsley
- 2 tablespoons chopped fresh mint
- 2 tablespoons extra virgin olive oil
- 1 tablespoon lemon juice
- 1 clove garlic, minced
- Salt and pepper to taste
- Crumbled feta cheese (optional)

Directions:

- In a large mixing bowl, combine chickpeas, cherry tomatoes, cucumber, red onion, parsley, and mint.
- In a small bowl, whisk together extra virgin olive oil, lemon juice, minced garlic, salt, and pepper to make the dressing.

- Pour the dressing over the chickpea mixture and toss until well coated.
- Taste and adjust seasoning as needed.
- Serve the Mediterranean Chickpea Salad chilled or at room temperature, garnished with crumbled feta cheese if desired.

Nutrition Facts (per serving):

- Calories: 248
- Fat: 10g
- Saturated Fat: 1g
- Cholesterol: 0mg
- Sodium: 262mg
- Carbohydrate: 31g
- Protein: 9g
- Fiber: 8g
- Calcium: 84mg
- Iron: 3mg

Potassium: 464mg

Prep Time: 10 mins

Total Time: 10 mins

Servings: 4

4. Turkey and Avocado Wrap

Ingredients:

- 4 whole-grain tortillas
- 8 oz sliced turkey breast
- 1 ripe avocado, sliced
- 1 cup mixed greens (such as spinach, arugula, or lettuce)
- 1/4 cup diced tomatoes
- 1/4 cup diced red onion
- 2 tablespoons Greek yogurt (optional)
- 1 tablespoon Dijon mustard (optional)
- Salt and pepper to taste

Directions:

- Lay out the whole-grain tortillas on a clean surface.
- Divide the sliced turkey breast evenly among the tortillas, placing it in the center of each tortilla.
- Top each tortilla with avocado slices, mixed greens, diced tomatoes, and diced red onion.
- If desired, spread Greek yogurt and Dijon mustard over the toppings for added flavor.
- Season with salt and pepper to taste.
- Fold the sides of each tortilla inward, then roll it up tightly to form a wrap.
- Slice the wraps in half diagonally before serving.

Nutrition Facts (per serving):

- Calories: 285
- Fat: 12g
- Saturated Fat: 2g
- Cholesterol: 45mg
- Sodium: 602mg
- Carbohydrate: 24g
- Protein: 20g
- Fiber: 6g
- Calcium: 65mg
- Iron: 2mg
- Potassium: 460mg

Prep Time: 10 mins

Total Time: 10 mins

Servings: 4

5. Quinoa Stuffed Bell Peppers

Ingredients:

- 4 large bell peppers (any color), halved and seeds removed
- 1 cup cooked quinoa
- 1 can (15 oz) black beans, drained and rinsed
- 1 cup diced tomatoes

- 1/2 cup corn kernels (fresh, frozen, or canned)
- 1/4 cup diced red onion
- 2 cloves garlic, minced
- 1 teaspoon ground cumin
- 1/2 teaspoon chili powder
- Salt and pepper to taste
- 1/4 cup chopped fresh cilantro
- 1/4 cup shredded cheddar cheese (optional)

Directions:

- Preheat the oven to 375°F (190°C). Arrange the halved bell peppers in a baking dish, cut side up.
- In a large mixing bowl, combine cooked quinoa, black beans, diced tomatoes, corn kernels, red onion, minced garlic, ground cumin, chili powder, salt, pepper, and chopped cilantro. Mix well.
- Spoon the quinoa mixture evenly into each bell pepper half, pressing down gently to pack it in.
- Cover the baking dish with aluminum foil and bake in the preheated oven for 25-30 minutes, or until the bell peppers are tender.
- If using shredded cheddar cheese, sprinkle it over the stuffed bell peppers during the last 5 minutes of baking, then return to the oven until the cheese is melted and bubbly.

- Remove from the oven and let cool slightly before serving.

Nutrition Facts (per serving, 1 stuffed pepper half):

- Calories: 170
- Fat: 1.5g
- Saturated Fat: 0.5g
- Cholesterol: 3mg
- Sodium: 290mg
- Carbohydrate: 32g
- Protein: 8g
- Fiber: 7g
- Calcium: 60mg
- Iron: 2mg

Potassium: 526mg

Prep Time: 15 mins

Total Time: 45 mins

Servings: 8 (2 stuffed pepper halves per serving)

Dinner Recipes

1. Baked Lemon Herb Salmon

Ingredients:

- 4 salmon fillets (about 6 oz each)
- 2 tablespoons olive oil
- 2 cloves garlic, minced
- 1 teaspoon lemon zest
- 2 tablespoons lemon juice
- 1 tablespoon chopped fresh parsley
- 1 tablespoon chopped fresh dill
- Salt and pepper to taste
- Lemon slices for garnish

Directions:

- Preheat the oven to 375°F (190°C). Lightly grease a baking dish with olive oil or cooking spray.
- Place the salmon fillets in the prepared baking dish.
- In a small bowl, whisk together olive oil, minced garlic, lemon zest, lemon juice, chopped parsley, chopped dill, salt, and pepper.
- Pour the lemon herb mixture over the salmon fillets, making sure they are evenly coated.
- Arrange lemon slices on top of each salmon fillet for additional flavor.
- Bake in the preheated oven for 12-15 minutes, or until the salmon is cooked through and flakes easily with a fork.

- Remove from the oven and let the salmon rest for a few minutes before serving.

Nutrition Facts (per serving):

- Calories: 320
- Fat: 20g
- Saturated Fat: 3.5g
- Cholesterol: 80mg
- Sodium: 150mg
- Carbohydrate: 1g
- Protein: 34g
- Fiber: 0g
- Calcium: 38mg
- Iron: 1mg
- Potassium: 710mg

Prep Time: 10 mins

Total Time: 25 mins

Servings: 4

2. Vegetable Stir-Fry with Tofu

Ingredients:

- 1 block (14 oz) firm tofu, drained and cubed
- 2 tablespoons soy sauce

- 1 tablespoon sesame oil
- 1 tablespoon cornstarch
- 2 tablespoons olive oil
- 2 cloves garlic, minced
- 1 tablespoon grated fresh ginger
- 1 bell pepper, thinly sliced
- 1 cup broccoli florets
- 1 carrot, julienned
- 1 cup snap peas
- 1/4 cup low-sodium vegetable broth
- 2 tablespoons hoisin sauce
- Cooked brown rice or quinoa for serving

Directions:

- In a bowl, combine cubed tofu, soy sauce, sesame oil, and cornstarch. Toss gently to coat the tofu evenly.
- Heat olive oil in a large skillet or wok over medium-high heat. Add minced garlic and grated ginger, and sauté for 1 minute until fragrant.
- Add tofu to the skillet and cook until golden brown on all sides, about 5-7 minutes. Remove tofu from the skillet and set aside.

- In the same skillet, add bell pepper, broccoli, carrot, and snap peas. Stir-fry for 5-6 minutes until vegetables are tender-crisp.
- Return tofu to the skillet, and add vegetable broth and hoisin sauce. Cook for another 2-3 minutes, stirring occasionally, until the sauce thickens and coats the tofu and vegetables.
- Serve the vegetable stir-fry over cooked brown rice or quinoa.

Nutrition Facts (per serving, without rice or quinoa):

- Calories: 220
- Fat: 14g
- Saturated Fat: 2g
- Cholesterol: 0mg
- Sodium: 480mg
- Carbohydrate: 15g
- Protein: 12g
- Fiber: 4g
- Calcium: 130mg
- Iron: 3mg
- Potassium: 470mg

Prep Time: 15 mins

Total Time: 25 mins

Servings: 4

3. Lemon Herb Grilled Chicken

Ingredients:

- 4 boneless, skinless chicken breasts
- 2 tablespoons olive oil
- 2 cloves garlic, minced
- 1 teaspoon lemon zest
- 2 tablespoons lemon juice
- 1 tablespoon chopped fresh parsley
- 1 tablespoon chopped fresh thyme
- Salt and pepper to taste
- Lemon slices for garnish

Directions:

- In a small bowl, whisk together olive oil, minced garlic, lemon zest, lemon juice, chopped parsley, chopped thyme, salt, and pepper to make the marinade.
- Place the chicken breasts in a shallow dish or resealable plastic bag. Pour the marinade over the chicken, making sure it's evenly coated. Marinate in the refrigerator for at least 30 minutes, or up to 4 hours.

- Preheat the grill to medium-high heat. Remove the chicken from the marinade and discard any excess marinade.
- Grill the chicken breasts for 6-7 minutes per side, or until cooked through and no longer pink in the center. The internal temperature should reach 165°F (74°C).
- Remove from the grill and let the chicken rest for a few minutes before serving.
- Garnish with lemon slices and additional chopped herbs if desired.

Nutrition Facts (per serving):

- Calories: 240
- Fat: 10g
- Saturated Fat: 1.5g
- Cholesterol: 90mg
- Sodium: 180mg
- Carbohydrate: 2g
- Protein: 34g
- Fiber: 0g
- Calcium: 22mg
- Iron: 1mg
- Potassium: 490mg

Prep Time: 10 mins (plus marinating time)

Total Time: 30 mins

Servings: 4

4. Vegetarian Lentil Shepherd's Pie

Ingredients:

For the mashed potato topping:

- 4 large potatoes, peeled and cubed
- 2 tablespoons butter or olive oil
- 1/4 cup milk or vegetable broth
- Salt and pepper to taste

For the lentil filling:

- 1 cup dry green or brown lentils
- 2 cups vegetable broth
- 1 tablespoon olive oil
- 1 onion, diced
- 2 carrots, diced
- 2 celery stalks, diced
- 2 cloves garlic, minced
- 1 teaspoon dried thyme
- 1 teaspoon dried rosemary
- 1 cup frozen peas

- Salt and pepper to taste

Directions:

- Preheat the oven to 375°F (190°C).
- In a large pot, bring the lentils and vegetable broth to a boil. Reduce heat to low, cover, and simmer for 20-25 minutes, or until the lentils are tender and most of the liquid is absorbed.
- While the lentils are cooking, place the peeled and cubed potatoes in a separate pot and cover with water. Bring to a boil and cook until tender, about 15 minutes.
- Drain the potatoes and mash them with butter or olive oil, milk or vegetable broth, salt, and pepper until smooth. Set aside.
- In a large skillet, heat olive oil over medium heat. Add diced onion, carrots, celery, and minced garlic. Cook until vegetables are softened, about 5-7 minutes.
- Stir in cooked lentils, dried thyme, dried rosemary, frozen peas, salt, and pepper. Cook for an additional 5 minutes, until the peas are heated through.
- Transfer the lentil filling to a baking dish and spread the mashed potatoes evenly over the top.

- Bake in the preheated oven for 25-30 minutes, or until the mashed potatoes are lightly golden on top.
- Remove from the oven and let it cool for a few minutes before serving.

Nutrition Facts (per serving):

- Calories: 320
- Fat: 6g
- Saturated Fat: 2g
- Cholesterol: 10mg
- Sodium: 480mg
- Carbohydrate: 54g
- Protein: 15g
- Fiber: 11g
- Calcium: 67mg
- Iron: 5mg
- Potassium: 1234mg

Prep Time: 20 mins

Total Time: 1 hour 15 mins

Servings: 6

5. Baked Spaghetti Squash with Tomato Basil Sauce

Ingredients:

For the spaghetti squash:

- 1 medium spaghetti squash
- 1 tablespoon olive oil
- Salt and pepper to taste

For the tomato basil sauce:

- 2 tablespoons olive oil
- 2 cloves garlic, minced
- 1 can (14 oz) crushed tomatoes
- 1/4 cup chopped fresh basil
- 1 teaspoon dried oregano
- Salt and pepper to taste

Directions:

- Preheat the oven to 400°F (200°C).
- Cut the spaghetti squash in half lengthwise and scoop out the seeds with a spoon. Drizzle the cut sides with olive oil and season with salt and pepper.
- Place the squash halves, cut side down, on a baking sheet lined with parchment paper. Roast in the preheated oven for 35-45 minutes, or until the squash is tender and easily pierced with a fork.
- While the squash is roasting, prepare the tomato basil sauce. In a saucepan, heat olive oil over

medium heat. Add minced garlic and cook until fragrant, about 1 minute.
- Stir in crushed tomatoes, chopped fresh basil, dried oregano, salt, and pepper. Simmer the sauce for 15-20 minutes, stirring occasionally, until it thickens slightly.
- Once the spaghetti squash is done roasting, remove it from the oven and let it cool slightly. Use a fork to scrape the flesh of the squash into strands.
- Serve the spaghetti squash topped with the tomato basil sauce. Garnish with additional fresh basil if desired.

Nutrition Facts (per serving):

- Calories: 120
- Fat: 7g
- Saturated Fat: 1g
- Cholesterol: 0mg
- Sodium: 370mg
- Carbohydrate: 14g
- Protein: 2g
- Fiber: 4g
- Calcium: 80mg
- Iron: 2mg

Potassium: 480mg

Prep Time: 10 mins

Total Time: 50 mins

Servings: 4

Snack Recipes

1. Greek Yogurt with Berries and Almonds

Ingredients:

- 1 cup plain Greek yogurt
- 1/2 cup mixed berries (such as strawberries, blueberries, raspberries)
- 1 tablespoon sliced almonds
- 1 teaspoon honey (optional)

Directions:

- Spoon Greek yogurt into a serving bowl.
- Top with mixed berries and sliced almonds.
- Drizzle with honey if desired.
- Serve immediately or refrigerate until ready to eat.

Nutrition Facts (per serving):

- Calories: 180
- Fat: 6g

- Saturated Fat: 0.5g
- Cholesterol: 10mg
- Sodium: 40mg
- Carbohydrate: 17g
- Protein: 15g
- Fiber: 3g
- Calcium: 200mg
- Iron: 1mg

Potassium: 250mg

Prep Time: 5 mins

Total Time: 5 mins

Servings: 1

2. Avocado Toast with Tomato and Basil

Ingredients:

- 1 ripe avocado
- 2 slices whole-grain bread, toasted
- 1 small tomato, sliced
- 2-3 fresh basil leaves, chopped
- Salt and pepper to taste
- Red pepper flakes (optional)

Directions:

- Halve the avocado, remove the pit, and scoop the flesh into a bowl. Mash the avocado with a fork until smooth.
- Spread mashed avocado evenly onto the toasted whole-grain bread slices.
- Top each avocado toast with sliced tomatoes and chopped basil leaves.
- Season with salt, pepper, and red pepper flakes if desired.
- Serve immediately.

Nutrition Facts (per serving):

- Calories: 250
- Fat: 15g
- Saturated Fat: 2g
- Cholesterol: 0mg
- Sodium: 200mg
- Carbohydrate: 25g
- Protein: 6g
- Fiber: 8g
- Calcium: 50mg
- Iron: 2mg
- Potassium: 700mg

Prep Time: 5 mins

Total Time: 5 mins

Servings: 1

3. Cucumber and Hummus Sandwiches

Ingredients:

- 1 medium cucumber, thinly sliced
- 4 slices whole-grain bread
- 1/2 cup hummus
- 1 tablespoon chopped fresh dill (optional)
- Salt and pepper to taste

Directions:

- Lay out the whole-grain bread slices on a clean surface.
- Spread a generous layer of hummus onto each bread slice.
- Arrange thinly sliced cucumber rounds on top of two bread slices.
- Sprinkle chopped fresh dill over the cucumber slices if desired, and season with salt and pepper.
- Place the remaining bread slices on top to form sandwiches.
- Cut each sandwich in half diagonally.

- Serve immediately, or wrap in parchment paper or plastic wrap for later.

Nutrition Facts (per serving):

- Calories: 250
- Fat: 10g
- Saturated Fat: 1g
- Cholesterol: 0mg
- Sodium: 400mg
- Carbohydrate: 34g
- Protein: 9g
- Fiber: 8g
- Calcium: 110mg
- Iron: 2mg
- Potassium: 540mg

Prep Time: 10 mins

Total Time: 10 mins

Servings: 2

4. Energy Bites

Ingredients:

- 1 cup rolled oats
- 1/2 cup natural peanut butter

- 1/4 cup honey or maple syrup
- 1/4 cup ground flaxseed
- 1/4 cup mini chocolate chips or raisins
- 1 teaspoon vanilla extract
- Pinch of salt

Directions:

- In a large mixing bowl, combine rolled oats, peanut butter, honey or maple syrup, ground flaxseed, chocolate chips or raisins, vanilla extract, and a pinch of salt.
- Stir well until all ingredients are fully combined.
- Using clean hands, roll the mixture into small balls, about 1 inch in diameter.
- Place the energy bites on a baking sheet lined with parchment paper.
- Refrigerate the energy bites for at least 30 minutes to firm up.
- Once firm, transfer the energy bites to an airtight container and store them in the refrigerator for up to one week.

Nutrition Facts (per serving, about 2 energy bites):

- Calories: 200
- Fat: 10g

- Saturated Fat: 2g
- Cholesterol: 0mg
- Sodium: 50mg
- Carbohydrate: 24g
- Protein: 6g
- Fiber: 4g
- Calcium: 40mg
- Iron: 1.5mg
- Potassium: 180mg

Prep Time: 10 mins

Total Time: 40 mins (including chilling time)

Servings: 12 (about 24 energy bites)

5. Apple Slices with Almond Butter

Ingredients:

- 2 medium apples, cored and sliced
- 1/4 cup almond butter
- 2 tablespoons chopped almonds
- Cinnamon (optional)

Directions:

- Arrange the apple slices on a serving plate.
- Place almond butter in a small bowl for dipping.

- Sprinkle chopped almonds over the almond butter.
- Optionally, dust the apple slices with cinnamon for added flavor.
- Serve the apple slices with almond butter and enjoy!

Nutrition Facts (per serving):

- Calories: 220
- Fat: 12g
- Saturated Fat: 1g
- Cholesterol: 0mg
- Sodium: 5mg
- Carbohydrate: 28g
- Protein: 5g
- Fiber: 7g
- Calcium: 80mg
- Iron: 1.5mg
- Potassium: 400mg

Prep Time: 5 mins

Total Time: 5 mins

Servings: 2

CONCLUSION

In conclusion, the EPI diet, tailored for individuals with Exocrine Pancreatic Insufficiency, emphasizes nutrient-dense foods to support optimal digestion and overall health. Throughout our discussion, we've explored various meal plans and recipes suitable for the EPI diet, ranging from breakfast to dinner, and even snacks.

We began by understanding EPI and its impact on digestive function, emphasizing the importance of selecting foods that are easily digestible and nutrient-rich. Next, we delved into the basics of the EPI diet, including calculating caloric needs and determining macronutrient ratios to ensure balanced nutrition.

Our exploration continued with meal planning strategies, providing guidelines for structuring meals and optimizing nutrient intake. We then presented beginner, intermediate, and advanced week meal plans, offering a variety of nutritious and delicious options for individuals following the EPI diet.

Additionally, we provided a diverse range of recipes suitable for the EPI diet, including breakfast options like Easy Fried Rice and Avocado Toast with Tomato and Basil, as well as lunch and dinner recipes such as Lentil Shepherd's Pie and Baked Lemon Herb Salmon.

For snacks, we offered quick and easy ideas like Energy Bites and Apple Slices with Almond Butter, providing convenient and satisfying options to help manage hunger between meals.

Overall, the EPI diet focuses on nourishing the body with wholesome, nutrient-dense foods while accommodating the specific needs of individuals with EPI. By incorporating these meal plans and recipes into their diet, individuals can support their digestive health and overall well-being.

Printed in Great Britain
by Amazon